Lovely Lavender: The Many Applications and Uses of Lavender Essential Oil

by Rashelle Johnson

Disclaimer:

The information contained in this book is for general information purposes only. The statements contained herein have not been evaluated nor approved by the US Food and Drug Administration. This book is sold with the understanding the author and/or publisher is not giving medical advice, nor should the information contained in this book replace medical advice, nor is it intended to diagnose or treat any disease, illness or other medical condition. Always seek the advice of your physician or a qualified health provider prior to starting any new treatment or if you have any questions regarding a medical condition.

All recommendations contained herein are believed to be effective, but the effectiveness has not been evaluated and no guarantees are made or implied nor is any liability taken. Use essential oils at your own risk and never use them to treat ailments against the advice of a qualified medical professional.

While we endeavor to keep the information up to date and correct, we make no representations or warranties of any kind, express or implied, about the completeness, accuracy, reliability, suitability or availability with respect to the book or the information, products, services, or related graphics contained book for any purpose. Any reliance you place on such information is therefore strictly at your own risk.

The information contained herein should not be considered to be complete. There may be safety concerns not mentioned in the book that you need to be aware of. Consult with your doctor or physician prior to using any essential oil or aromatherapy treatment.

Dedication:

My love of lavender essential oil led me to write this book. I use lavender in almost everything. I'd like to thank my ever-understanding friends and family members who were hit with a constant barrage of lavender products and oil blends in the days leading up to the writing of this book. Thanks for being there for me guys!

Contents

What is Lavender?

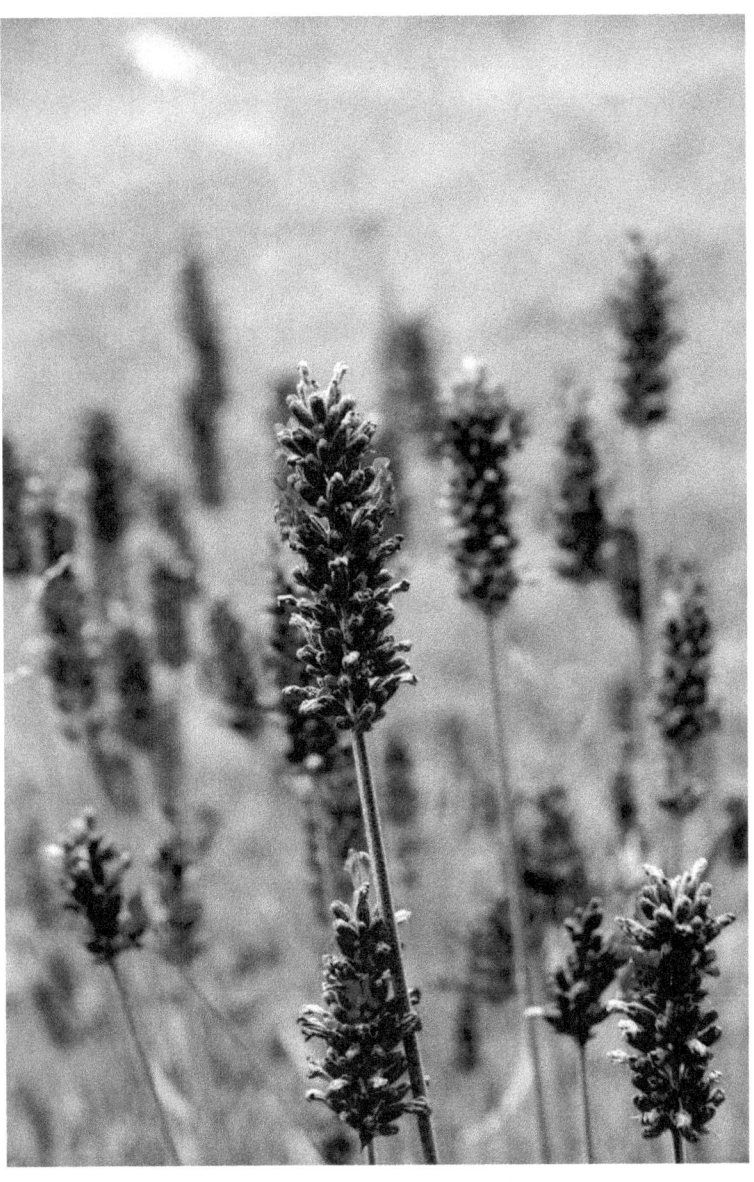

The lavender plant, or lavandula, as it's scientifically known, is a pretty flowering plant native to Europe, Africa and the Mediterranean. There are 39 different species of lavandula known to exist today, the most common of which is Lavandula angustfolia, also known as English lavender or common lavender. When we use the term "lavender" in this book, this is the species of lavandula being referenced.

Lavender is grown commercially and in gardens all over the world. To those familiar with the plant, the long stalks and purple flower clusters at its top are instantly recognizable. Lavender is a popular choice for gardeners because it's easy to grow and doesn't require perfect soil or a lot of water. In fact, lavender thrives in dry, rocky habitats and is well-known for its drought-resistant qualities.

Those familiar with the smoky floral smell of lavender oil will probably be surprised to hear lavender is a member of the mint family. While some lavender oils do have a hint of mint in the fragrance, lavender has a smoky floral note that gives way to a slightly campherous fragrance. The smell of lavender is somewhat of an acquired taste, but most people come to love it. Being an author of a book extolling the virtues of lavender oil, I'm almost embarrassed to admit I didn't like the smell at first. I bought some lavender oil, opened the bottle once and smelled it, then tossed the bottle in the cupboard for a couple months. I rediscovered it while looking for something else in the cupboard. On a whim, I opened the bottle and took another whiff. It smelled much better the second time around and I was hooked.

There are a number of uses for lavender. Traditionally, it was used in baths for its scent and because it was thought to purify the body and the mind. It has also seen use as an herb that's been added to food and drinks and as an air freshener that can be dried and left sitting in a room to make it smell clean and fresh. The scent of lavender is both soothing and sedative, making it a popular choice for those looking to wind down after a long, hard day.

Here are just some of the many ways lavender is used today:

- Acne control.
- Added to bath water.
- Added to clothes dryer.
- Antibiotic.
- Burn treatment.
- Calming and soothing frayed nerves.
- Circulation.
- Decoration.
- Depression.
- Fragrance.
- Grown in ornamental gardens.
- Hair loss.
- Headaches.
- Ingested in a number of culinary dishes.
- Insect repellent.
- Insomnia.
- Made into a calming tea.
- Made into essential oil.
- Made into honey or sugar.

- Massage oil.
- Pharmaceutical products.
- Potpourri.
- Promotes feelings of well-being.
- Relaxation.
- Sedative.
- Turned into ink.
- Used in a burner.

The many uses of lavender as an herb, a flower and as an essential oil has led some to call it the Swiss Army Knife of the plant world. The best part is it's all-natural and is safe for most people to use.

The History of Lavender

The documented use of lavender dates back to ancient Egypt, where lavender was used in perfumes and as a cure-all for many ailments and maladies. The rags used to wrap mummies were dipped in lavender prior to the mummification process. There have been pots and urns found in the tombs of ancient Egyptian royalty that still have the faint scent of lavender oil.

While the science behind why lavender worked wasn't understood until modern times, it didn't take long for our ancestors to figure out its therapeutic benefits. In ancient Greece, it was used for everything from relaxation to soothing the mentally insane. During the times of the Roman Empire, lavender was a highly-sought after fragrance. Petals were added to baths and the rich would add it to their smoking blends and smoke it in pipes. In fact, the word lavender is derived from the Latin word "lavare," which means to bathe. The Romans used it to scent everything, from their clothes to their bedding. Roman soldiers even carried it with them into battle and used it for first aid purposes. It's thought that it was the Romans who brought lavender to much of Europe as they invaded and conquered distant lands.

When the Great Plague hit Britain in the 17th century, people turned to lavender as a way to ward it off. It quickly became obvious that those working in the lavender fields were less prone to catching the plague and before long people began tying a sprig of lavender to each of their wrists. It's now known that lavender repels bugs. Since the plague was largely spread by infected fleas, this preventative measure may have saved the lives of large numbers of people who chose to wear lavender.

King, queens and all sorts of royalty were known for their marked appreciation of lavender. Cleopatra is said to have worn it as a perfume. Queen Elizabeth I demanded that fresh lavender flowers be available to her whenever she so desired and both her and Queen Elizabeth II used products made by Yardley and Co., which specialized in lavender-infused wares. King Charles VI of France has his bedding filled with lavender. You'd be hard-pressed to find royalty that didn't use lavender in one form or the other.

Lavender was brought to America by the first English colonists. The Shakers grew it commercially and sold it for a profit. Fast-forward to World War II, and lavender was used as an antiseptic by medics seeking to disinfect the wounds of soldiers.

Lavender essential oil is largely responsible for the popularity of aromatherapy and essential oils today. Shortly after the turn of the 20th century, scientist Rene Gattefosse was experimenting in his lab when he badly burnt his hand. It just so happened that a container of lavender essential oil was sitting nearby and he dipped his hand in it to ease the pain. To his amazement, the pain subsided almost immediately and his hand rapidly healed, leaving nary a scar or mark behind. It was this discovery that led into further experimentation on lavender oil and is largely responsible for the resurgence in popularity of essential oils today.

If essential oils were a family, lavender essential oil would be the patriarch of the family, overseeing a huge brood of other oils. Lavender oil is the most-used oil today and is popular amongst aromatherapists and perfumists alike.

Lavender Essential Oil

Lavender essential oil is oil distilled from the flower spikes of the lavender plant. It's the aromatic essence of the plant. When you smell a field of lavender, the fragrance that teases your nose is that of the oil contained within the flowers. The most common type of lavender essential oil comes from the Lavandula angustifolia plant. Every time you see lavender essential oil referred to, it's safe to assume it's from the Lavandula angustifolia plant.

There are numerous top 10 lists in books, magazine and on the Internet that list favorite essentials oils. Lavender essential oil is a top choice on almost every single one of these lists. You'd be hard-pressed to find a top 10 favorite oils list that doesn't have lavender somewhere on the list— and it's usually in the number one position. Most aromatherapists would agree it's one of the most versatile and capable essential oils there is.

The most common means of extracting lavender essential oil from the flowers of the plant is through steam distillation. The flowers are placed in a still full of water and brought to a boil. Steam that consists of water and essential oil rises to the top of the still and makes its way through a cooling coil. As it cools, it condenses back into liquid form. The essential oil is lighter than the water, so it rises to the top, where it can be separated out. The thin film on top of the water is almost pure essential oil.

There's always a little bit of oil left behind in the water. This oil/water mixture is used to create a product called a hydrosol, which smells like lavender, but doesn't offer the same health benefits as the essential oil does. Don't be fooled into thinking it's the same thing.

It's rare with lavender oils, but you may come across oils that have been extracted using solvents. Steer clear of these oils. Chemical solvents are used to pull the oils from the plants. The solvents are allowed to evaporate, leaving behind a hard substance called a concrete. The oils are then extracted from the concrete. When alcohol is used in the process, the result is lavender absolute. You want to steer clear of solvent-extracted oils because there's a significant amount of solvent left behind. The solvent extraction method isn't as common with lavender as it is with other floral oils because lavender oil is abundant in the flowers and is easy to extract via steam distillation.

Steam-distilled lavender essential oil is one of the safest essential oils sold today. While, as with any plant oil, there are people who do react negatively to it, those people are few and far between. It's one of the more gentle oils, and it's one of the few that many people feel comfortable applying topically undiluted. I don't recommend this practice because of the oil's high linalyl acetate content, but a lot of people swear by this method of topical application.

When you purchase lavender essential oil, it's important you make sure you're getting pure high-quality oil. Don't fall for the marketing gimmicks from companies claiming to have "certified" or "therapeutic-grade" oils. Essential oils are largely unregulated and any company making this claim is doing their own certification. If you're from the United States, there is no central agency or business group that ensures oils meet a certain standard. It's up to the individual company to determine what level of quality control they have.

Steer clear of absolutes and floral waters, because they don't have the same therapeutic values as essential oil does. Absolutes can contain solvents and other chemicals that can be detrimental to your health. Floral waters are good for their fragrance, but that's about it. Synthetic fragrances are the same thing. They're made in a lab and smell similar to lavender, but don't have the same chemical composition as essential oil.

Even 100% pure oils can vary in quality from manufacturer to manufacturer. Your best bet is to get your oil from a well-known company that's trusted by aromatherapists. Buy your oil from your local big-box retailer and you're sure to be disappointed. The best oils are grown and distilled under tightly controlled conditions. They cost more than the cheap stuff, but are well worth the extra money because they are consistent from batch to batch and will have similar qualities every time you use them.

Composition of Lavender Essential Oil

Lavender essential oil has as many as a couple hundred different naturally-occurring chemical components that act together to improve your health. Let's take a look at some of the most important constituents. Don't worry; you aren't going to need a degree in biochemistry to understand this section. I'll try to keep it as simple as possible.

The percentage breakdowns in this chapter are best-guess estimates as to how much of each compound is found in lavender essential oil. There are a number of variables that can affect how much of each compound makes it into the final product, so it's impossible to give exact numbers. The percentages can vary from supplier to supplier and even from batch to batch.

Beta-carophylene

This anti-inflammatory agent makes up nearly 5% of the chemical composition of lavender essential oil. It helps the body ward off inflammation, which is the main reason for a number of illnesses and ailments.

Camphor

The camphor content in lavender oil can be as high as 10% depending on the type of lavender used. Camphor has a cooling effect and is good for knocking down stubborn coughs. It can be a dermal and mucous membrane irritant in large amounts, so steer clear of oils high in camphor.

Eucalyptol

Some types of lavender oil contain eucalyptol, which has a powerful campherous fragrance. It's used to treat respiratory conditions and is analgesic when applied topically. Lavender essential oil made from spike lavender plants can contain as high as 20% eucalyptol content.

Linalool

Linalool is related to linalyl acetate in that it's required for the acetate to form. This close sibling of linalyl acetate makes up somewhere in the neighborhood of 30% of lavender oil. Linalool is thought to relieve stress while improving the manner in which the body responds to stressful situations. It's also believed to provide relief from a number of conditions, from headaches to insomnia. Some lab tests have even shown linalool to inhibit certain types of cancer from replicating.

Linalyl Acetate

Lavender essential oil contains just over 30% linalyl acetate. This chemical compound is found in a number of plants, namely spices and flowers. It's one of the main constituents of lavender oil. Linalyl acetate has a sedative effect and is one of the chemicals in lavender oil that helps you relax. It's believed to be anti-inflammatory as well. Combined with linalool, linalyl acetate is largely responsible for the scent of lavender oil.

Linalyl acetate can cause allergic reactions in some people. At full strength, it can be a strong dermal irritant.

This propensity for irritating the skin is dulled in the essential oil and skin reactions are rare.

Myrcene

Myrcene is present in lavender oil, but only in trace amounts. Myrcene is used as a decongestant and is capable of relieving mucus membrane discomfort when fragrances containing it are inhaled. Myrcene is also antiseptic and antiviral, but the small amount of myrcene in lavender oil probably renders this effect negligible.

Ocimene

There are two types of ocimene found in lavender essential oil and, between the two, they make up 6% - 8% of the oil. They are decongestant and have antibacterial, antiseptic and antiviral properties.

Pinene

Pinene is another compound good for respiratory health. It's mucolytic and is thought to be diuretic as well. It's also seen use as a tonic for rheumatism and other joint pain. There isn't a lot of pinene in lavender oil, but there's usually at least a little.

Terpinen-4-OL

Lavender oil contains just under 5 percent terpinen-4-OL content. This terpene is known for its germ-killing powers and is has strong antibacterial, antifungal and antiseptic properties.

Terpineol

Terpineol makes up less than one percent of the total chemical composition of lavender essential oil, but it has some interesting qualities. It's antibacterial and antiviral by nature and is considered to be a stimulant of the immune system. It's a warming component, but doesn't have much warming effect in lavender oil because it makes up so little of the total volume of the oil.

Keep in mind that these are just a few of the many beneficial chemicals found in lavender essential oil. There are hundreds of compounds that all work together to improve your health.

The Health Benefits of Lavender Oil

Lavender essential oil has a number of therapeutic properties. The properties discussed in this chapter are just some of the health benefits of lavender. Believe it or not, even though lavender has been in use for thousands of years, people are still finding new uses for it. It's one of the more versatile oils and has historically been used to treat almost anything you can imagine. Let's take a closer look at some of the health benefits of lavender oil.

Analgesic

When applied topically, lavender oil has been shown to relieve pain. It probably isn't going to make you completely forget about your aches and pains, but it might make them more tolerable. If you're looking strictly for pain relief, go with an oil that has stronger analgesic properties like wintergreen oil. If you're looking for the total package that helps you physically and emotionally deal with pain, lavender may fit the bill.

Anticonvulsant

Seizures are caused when the receptors in the brain start firing at a faster rate than they're supposed to. Lavender is said to slow down the firing of these electrical impulses, which in turn may help those who are prone to epileptic seizures. That said, there is anecdotal evidence that lavender may trigger seizures in some people. It may also interact with medications taken to reduce the risk of seizures. Discuss your options with your physician before attempting to use lavender to help with seizures.

Antidepressant

A depressed person is plagued by deep feelings of sadness and/or despair. This is a chronic condition caused by a hormonal imbalance in the body. Lavender oil has been used for centuries to treat depression. Recent clinical trials have shown it to be effective in easing depression in some people. If you're clinically depressed, seek immediate medical attention if your mood worsens or you start thinking of self-harm. Consult with your doctor before attempting to treat depression with lavender oil.

Antifungal

Lavender oil is antifungal, making it a good treatment for fungal infections like athlete's foot and yeast infections. Mix lavender oil with tea tree oil and dilute it heavily befor application for best results.

Anti-inflammatory

Inflammation is a common problem both inside and outside the body. Lavender oil fights inflammation and can help swelling go down. It's capable of easing the effects of diseases like rheumatism that are caused by inflammation and can be used to soothe irritated and inflamed skin caused by cuts, burns, bruises and insect bites.

Antiseptic

An antiseptic compound is one that prevents the growth of microorganisms that cause infection and disease.

Lavender essential oil contains a number of antiseptic compounds that seek and destroy harmful bacteria.

Antispasmodic

Looking for a way to ease the pain associated with muscle cramping? Lavender essential oil is antispasmodic, which means it can help relax muscles and relieve cramps. This property also means it's effective in helping with coughing that's caused by a spasmodic reaction.

Antiviral

The high linalool content in lavender oil makes it strongly antiviral. Lavender oil can be used as a preventative measure against viruses and experts suggest it's able to bolster the immune system to protect against the flu and other viral infections.

Carminative

A carminative substance is one that prevents gas. Lavender oil contains compounds that are known to be carminative by nature.

Cholagogue

Here's one you may not have heard of before. A cholagogue is a substance thought to promote the flow of bile from the liver. This helps with the digestive process and cleanses the liver. Lavender oil is said to have cholagogue properties.

Cicatrisant

Here's another term most people aren't familiar with. A cicatrisant agent helps wounds heal by promoting the formation of scar tissue. If you have a wound or damaged skin, lavender oil's cicatrisant properties can help it heal and may even help fade the scar away.

Cytophlactic

Lavender essential oil has cytophlactic properties, meaning it helps promote the formation of new cells. This is especially beneficially to aging or damaged skin when the oil is applied topically because it helps to keep the skin healthy.

Decongestant

Lavender essential oil can be used to provide cold and flu relief because of its decongestant properties. Fill up your sink with steaming hot water and put 4 to 5 drops of lavender oil in the water and stir it up. Place a damp towel over your head and hold your face over the sink, so that you're breathing in the steam rising off the water. It will help to break up any congestion you have. For a more effective treatment, try adding a few drops of eucalyptus oil to the water as well.

Deodorant

Store-bought deodorant is full of chemicals you shouldn't be putting anywhere near your body. Lavender oil is a natural deodorant that gets rid of odors. You can use it to replace your deodorant and you can use it as a natural air freshener. It's good at getting rid of bad smells no matter where they're found at.

Diuretic

A diuretic compound is one that causes the body to excrete water in the form of urine. Medicinal diuretics are used to treat a number of conditions like high blood pressure and hypertension. Lavender essential oil contains substances that are thought to be diuretic by nature.

Emmenagogue

Women can use emmenagogue oils like lavender oil to stimulate blood flow during menstruation. Because lavender oil has emmenagogue properties, it should be avoided by women who are pregnant.

Nervine

A nervine substance is one that helps the nervous system in some way. Lavender oil is thought to stimulate and strengthen the nervous system. If you've been feeling frazzled and stressed out, lavender essential oil may be just what you need to bring your body back into alignment. It can also help with anxiety and stress.

Rubifacient

Applying a rubifacient substance to your skin causes it to take on a slight red hue as the capillaries dilate and blood flow increases. Rubifacient compounds are often used to help alleviate pain associated with inflammation like that of osteoarthritis. Lavender essential oil is mildly rubifacient.

Sedative

The sedative properties of lavender essential oil help the body relax and wind down. This makes lavender a good choice for a warm bath at the end of the day. It also makes lavender a good choice for those suffering from insomnia.

Sudorific

Sudorific compounds promote sweating. This helps the body purge toxins through the sweat glands.

Vulnerary

Lavender oil contains chemical constituents that make it a good vulnerary compound. When it's used on wounds, it promotes healing. Lavender oil works especially well on minor burns.

Topical Application

Topical application of lavender oil is one of the best methods of delivering lavender oil to the body. Apply pure lavender essential oil to your skin and it will absorb almost immediately. The oil enters your blood stream and the helpful chemical constituents are spread throughout your entire body.

Neat application of lavender oil involves applying undiluted oil directly to the skin. There are numerous books and articles that state lavender essential oil is safe to apply neat. I'm of the opinion that it's probably safe for the vast majority of people when you only apply a few drops of undiluted oil to the skin, but I don't recommend this practice because it isn't safe for everyone. There are some people who can have a severe negative reaction to lavender oil. Skin sensitization can occur that could make your skin not only react negatively to lavender, but to any essential oil you apply in the future. People have applied lavender neat a single time and touched off a reaction that made them permanently allergic to lavender oil, even in diluted form. If you do decide to go against my advice and apply lavender essential oil neat, consult with your doctor and an aromatherapy professional first.

While it's relatively rare, there are some people who have a negative reaction to diluted oil. Always dilute new oil heavily and test it on a small area of skin prior to application to a larger area. Your best bet is to apply it and wait overnight to see if you have a reaction. Don't trust that lavender oil is completely safe just because you read it somewhere. There are a number of people out there who can attest to the fact that lavender oil can indeed cause irritation and skin sensitization. It isn't likely, but it is possible.

Diluted Application

Your best bet is to dilute your lavender oil with carrier oil prior to application. There are a number of carrier oils that can be used, the most common of which are sweet almond oil, Grapeseed oil and apricot kernel oil. Add 3 to 5 drops of lavender essential oil to a teaspoon of one of these carrier oils and you'll be ready to apply your lavender oil topically in one of the safest ways possible. When you use carrier oil, you get the added health benefit of the carrier oil along with the essential oil you're using.

To apply an oil blend to your body, place a few drops on the area of application and rub or massage it into the skin. When you massage it into the skin, you get the added relaxation and muscle pain relief of the massage in addition to the therapeutic qualities of the oil.

Here are a few carrier oils and the health benefits you can reap from them:

Sweet Almond Oil

This popular oil nourishes the skin and works well for massage oil.

Apricot Kernel Oil

This is light oil is good for dry and chapped skin. It promotes the healing of damaged skin.

Avocado Oil

Works well for dry and chapped skin because it contains a lot of vitamins and moisture. Avocado oil should be combined with other oils as part of an oil blend. For best results, use it as 10% of your oil blend.

Grapeseed Oil

This is a light oil that's good for all types of skin. It's ideal for use with essential oils because it doesn't have much scent. Be careful because it's extracted through use of solvents and can cause sensitization issues.

Hazelnut Oil

This is another light oil that works well as a massage oil. It works best for people who have oily skin.

Jojoba Oil

This is technically a liquid wax, but it's used in a manner similar to carrier oil. It has an extended shelf life and is similar in makeup to the sebum produced by the skin.

Olive Oil

This heavy oil is good for dry skin, but the strong smell can make olive oil difficult to use in aromatherapy blends. It works well when creating salves and lotions that are applied to the skin for medical purposes.

Baths

There's nothing more relaxing than bathing or soaking yourself with water infused with lavender essential oil. The most direct way is to add 4 to 8 drops of lavender oil to the tub while it's filling. Let the tub fill and stir it up because the oil will rise to the top and tends to pool up. Soak in the tub for 10 to 15 minutes, agitating the water every few minutes to mix the lavender oil back into the water. When you get out of the tub there should be an oily sheen at the surface of the water. This oil will coat your skin as you rise from the tub, leaving you smelling fresh and feeling relaxed.

Another way of applying the oil to your entire body is to place 10 to 20 drops in a Jacuzzi or hot tub. The swirling water will keep the oil blended in and will apply it to the entire submerged portion of your body. You get the added bonus of having a great smelling hot tub that's free of bacteria and fungus.

You can do the same thing in the shower, but it's going to take a little more work. Dilute your lavender oil with carrier oil and place the mixture on a washcloth or small towel. Rub the cloth all over your body as you let the water from the shower wash over you. By the time the shower's done, you'll be relaxed and ready to unwind.

You can also soak your hands and feet in a bath filled with water and a few drops of oil. Add 5 drops of lavender oil to a washbasin big enough to fit both of your feet in and let them soak for up to a half hour. This is a great way to relax and can kill fungal infections like athlete's foot. Stir the water up frequently or use a dispersant for best results.

Compresses

Compresses can be created by adding 5 to 10 drops of oil to a bowl full of water and dipping a towel into it. Add the oil to the bowl and stir it up, then wait for the oil to rise to the top. When it does, use the towel to soak up the oil that's floating on the surface. Wring out any excess water and apply the compress to your body.

Cold compresses use cold water to relieve a number of conditions. Headaches, swelling and muscle aches and pains can all be relieved through use of cold compresses. Hot compresses use hot water and have a number of uses as well. You can use hot compresses to alleviate pain associated with arthritis, cramping, menstrual pain and a number of other aches and pains.

The most effective way to use compresses is to combine them with massage therapy. Massage diluted oil into the affected area and let it soak in a bit. Once the massage is done, apply a compress to the same area. When you combine compresses and massage therapy only use a few drops of essential oil in your compress. You've already massaged oil into the same location and you don't want to use too much.

Ingesting Lavender Oil

Lavender essential oil should not be consumed, unless it's done under strict medical supervision for a specific reason. For one, adding an essential oil to your diet is the least effective means of getting the oil into your body. Topical application and diffusion are much more effective and deliver the chemical compounds in the oil directly into your system without them having to pass through your digestive system, where they can be damaged and rendered worthless for all intents and purposes.

Ingesting essential oils is a dangerous game, and if you decide you want to add lavender oil to your diet, you should do so under the direct consent of your doctor and an aromatherapy professional. You may be better off consuming lavender tea, which is made from the dried flowers of the lavender plant. You'll still get some of the health benefits of the oil, but not in as high of a dosage as you would by ingesting lavender oil.

You may see recipes that call for lavender oil. These recipes generally aren't referring to essential oil. They're referring to lavender-infused oil that's made by soaking lavender flowers in olive or canola oil. You can make your own lavender cooking oil by picking or buying fresh lavender flowers and placing them into jars filled with olive oil. Seal the jars and let them sit in a cool, dark place for a month or two and you'll have lavender cooking oil. This is nowhere near as strong as adding a few drops of essential oil to cooking oil, so don't assume it's the same thing.

Consuming lavender essential oil can result in lavender poisoning. Blurry vision, cramping, shortness of breath and vomiting can all occur when lavender oil is ingested in unsafe amounts. If you or someone you know ingested lavender oil and is starting to show signs of distress, contact your local poison control hotline immediately. Getting help as soon as possible is critical when lavender poisoning is a concern.

The Many Faces of Diffusion

Another great way of reaping the benefits of lavender oil is to diffuse it into a room. Diffusion is the process of breaking essential oil up into tiny particles and spreading the fragrance throughout a room. The compounds in the oils enter your bloodstream through your lungs and through blood vessels in your nasal passage. Diffusing lavender oil into a room isn't just good for your body; it also freshens the air and kills airborne pathogens.

There are a number of ways to diffuse lavender oil, some of which can be done for free using items you probably already own. If you have the money and are serious about aromatherapy, you can invest in electronic diffusers that disperse oil throughout the room efficiently and quietly.

There are two basic types of diffusion: hot and cold. Hot diffusion uses methods that warm the oil to disperse it into a room. Cold methods don't heat the oil before dispersing it. With hot diffusion, there's the potential of damaging the aromatic compounds in the oil and rendering them ineffective. Cold methods are preferable to hot or warm methods. We'll cover both hot and cold methods in this chapter. While cold methods are the preferred method for insuring oils are undamaged after diffusion, hot methods are still in use.

Candles

The heat of a candle can be used to disperse essential oil into a room. This can be done by melting the candle wax and adding a few drops of oil directly to the wax or by placing the candle under a ceramic container that holds lavender oil mixed with water. As the oil heats up, the fragrance is spread through the room.

Electric Fan Diffuser

An electric fan diffuser blows cool air across the top of a tray or pad containing your oil. As the air passed the tray, it picks up the fragrance and carries it out into the room. Fan diffusers come in various sizes. The larger diffusers are capable of diffusing oil into a large room, but they tend to be rather loud.

Electric Heat Diffuser

This hot method of diffusion uses a heating grid to warm up a reservoir containing oil and water. The heat slowly releases the scent of the oil. The nice thing about electric methods is you can set them on a timer so oil is only diffused when you want it to be.

Lamp Diffusers

A lamp diffuser is made of a ring that fits around a regular light bulb. As the light bulb heats up, the oil in the ring heats up and is dispersed into the room. This method doesn't work with high efficiency bulbs and has fallen out of favor in the last few years.

Nebulizer

Nebulizers are one of the more expensive forms of diffusion. They're also one of the most effective. A nebulizer works by vaporizing essential oil and dispersing atom-sized particles of oil into the room. They're capable of dispersing oil into large rooms that render other diffusion methods ineffective. This is the preferred method of diffusion for most professional aromatherapists. The only downside is nebulizers tend to be a bit on the loud side. As long as you can deal with the noise, a nebulizer is the way to go.

Reed Diffusers

A reed diffuser consists of a small pot with a number of wood reeds in it. Oil is placed in the pot and it travels up the reeds, diffusing fragrance as it moves up the reed. This method is most effective in small rooms.

Steam

Bring 3 cups of water to a running boil. Add the water to a bowl and add 5 to 10 drops of lavender oil while the water is still steaming. The steam will carry the oil with it as it evaporates into the room. This method doesn't last long, but all it costs you is a few cups of water.

Terra Cotta

Oil is placed inside a small pot or pendant that's made of porous material. The oil slowly seeps through the pot and the smell permeates the room. These porous pots can make a small room smell great for weeks on end.

Tissue

This is one of the easiest methods of diffusion and it can be done for next to nothing. Add 5 to 10 drops of lavender oil to a tissue and walk around the room waving the tissue in the air, then set the tissue on a table or countertop out in the open. This method works well in small rooms.

25 Ways to Use Lavender Oil

There are a number of interesting and surprising ways you can use lavender oil. Here are 25 of them, in no particular order:

1. Dilute it and massage it into your skin right before bed time to combat insomnia. Add a couple drops to your pillow for a little extra help falling asleep.
2. Fill your sink with hot water and add lavender oil to the water. Place a towel over your head and place your face over the sink. Inhale the steam to break up mucus in both your sinuses and your chest. This will also help with allergies.
3. Insect repellent.
4. Add lavender oil to a warm foot bath and soak your feet in it to relieve stress.
5. Add a few drops of lavender oil to your dryer while drying your clothes to make them smell fresh and clean.
6. When you've been stung by a bee or bitten by a mosquito, rub a drop or two of oil onto the bite or sting to prevent swelling and to stop itching.
7. Rub diluted lavender oil into sunburnt skin to ease pain and promote healing.
8. Applying diluted lavender oil to an area where you're having acne trouble can kill the bacteria that are causing the acne flare-up.
9. Diluted lavender oil can be rubbed into your scalp to help alleviate dandruff.
10. Diffuse lavender oil at the end of a long day to help you relax.

11. Diffuse lavender oil to help with allergies.
12. Add lavender oil to the water you put in your steam iron to make your clothes smell good and keep them fresh.
13. Dilute lavender oil with carrier oil and massage it into sore muscles to relieve aches and pains.
14. Use lavender oil on a minor cut or scrape to promote healing and prevent infection. Dilute it with carrier oil prior to applying it to the wound.
15. Use lavender oil on a minor burn to promote healing and ease the pain.
16. When you have a headache, dilute lavender oil and rub it into your temples and the back of your neck to relieve the pain.
17. Rub diluted lavender oil into an area with scarring and the scar may start to fade away.
18. Mix lavender oil with carrier oil and use it on dry or damaged skin.
19. Rub a drop or two of lavender oil into each of your armpits to use it as a deodorant.
20. Rub a few drops of lavender oil into the bottoms of your feet to help you relax.
21. Massage diluted lavender oil into the area around your ears to help ease the pain associated with an ear infection.
22. Massage a few drops of lavender oil into your abdomen to relieve cramping associated with menstruation.
23. Dab a drop or two onto your wrists and use it as a great smelling perfume.
24. Massage a few drops of lavender oil into your hair to keep it smelling fresh and clean.

25. Diffuse it into the air to stimulate your appetite.

Making Your Own Lavender Essential Oil

Lavender essential oil is fairly easy to make yourself at home. Be aware that this method uses alcohol to pull the oil out of the lavender flowers and there may be trace amounts of alcohol left behind in your oil.

You're going to need the following items:

- The flowering buds of lavender plants. If you're feeling industrious, you can grow your own. If not, you can order them online. Some people buy them from a local florist or nursery, but you're going to pay a premium if you get them that way. If you buy them online, try to find organically grown buds.
- Vodka. The cheap stuff works fine.
- Mason jars.
- 3 coffee filters.
- A mortar and pestle.

Follow these steps to make your own lavender essential oil:

1. Crush the lavender buds using the mortar and pestle. You just want to crush them a bit. If you smash them too much, you're going to have a tough time extracting the oil.
2. Place the crushed buds into a mason jar.
3. Fill the jar with vodka until it's just over the top of the buds. Seal the jar tightly.

4. Shake the jar vigorously 3 times a day for 1 week.
5. Place a coffee filter over another mason jar and strain just the liquid into the jar. The liquid is made up of essential oil mixed with alcohol.
6. Set a coffee filter over the top of the jar and let it sit until the alcohol evaporates away, leaving behind the essential oil.
7. Filter the oil through a coffee filter one more time to get rid of any sediment.
8. Congrats! You now have homemade lavender essential oil.

NOTE: Be sure to store your lavender oil in a dark container. Bright light can damage your oil and degrade its quality.

Lavender Oil Recipes: Make Your Own Products with Lavender Oil

Lavender essential oil is one of the most popular and versatile essential oils available today. You can make a number of products and blends with it that cover everything from freshening the air to repelling insects. This is the chapter you bought the book for, folks. The recipes.

Air Freshener #1

Lavender air freshener will infuse your home with the scent of lavender while cleaning the air in the process. This air freshener combines the power of lavender oil with that of baking soda for a double whammy that stops bad smells in their tracks.

Ingredients

1 Mason jar (or any glass container with a metal lid)

½ cup baking soda

1 small nail

1 hammer

A handful of dried lavender buds

15 drops lavender essential oil

Directions

1. Add baking soda, dried lavender buds and the lavender essential oil to the Mason jar and place the lid on the jar.

2. Shake the jar up until the contents are thoroughly mixed.
3. Use the hammer and nail to poke 20 to 30 small holes in the lid of the jar.
4. Place your air freshener somewhere you want to infuse with the smell of lavender.

NOTE: Large rooms may require more than one air freshener. Try placing one in the center and one in each corner of the room.

Air Freshener #2

This air freshener can be sprayed in a room where you want to quickly get rid of bad smells—like the bathroom after the man of the house uses it. A few sprays of this air freshener will leave most rooms smelling clean and fresh.

Ingredients

1 cup water

5 drops lemon essential oil

10 drops lavender essential oil

A spray bottle.

Directions

1. Add water and essential oils to the spray bottle.
2. Shake up the mixture before you spray it because the oil will rise to the top over time.
3. Spray 2 to 3 sprays into the room you want to freshen.

Bath Fizzies

If you've never experienced a bath fizzie, you don't know what you're missing. You throw one in the tub with you and it bubbles and fizzes, releasing essential oils, carrier oils and great scents into the tub water. You could buy your bath fizzies commercially from any number of sources, but making them yourself is half the fun. This fizzy uses just lavender oil, but you can use any other oils you'd like.

The key to getting it to fizz properly is the baking soda and citric acid. Get those two items together and add water and it creates an interesting fizzing effect.

Ingredients

1 cup citric acid

2 cups baking soda

20 drops lavender essential oil

2 teaspoons dried lavender buds

Spray bottle filed with witch hazel.

Natural purple coloring.

Plastic molds.

Directions

1. Add the baking soda and citric acid to a small bowl and stir until completely blended.
2. Add ¼ teaspoon of natural purple coloring and mix it up. You can add a bit more if you want your fizzies to be a darker purple color, but don't

overdo it. You don't want to have to scrub purple dye off of your tub.

3. Add 20 drops of lavender essential oil. Slowly add the oil and stir it in a few drops at a time.

4. Add the lavender buds and stir into the mix.

5. Set the spray bottle to a fine mist and spray witch hazel on the mixture. As you spray it, stir it into the mixture.

6. Once the mixture is able to be molded and is able to stay in place, stop spraying and place the mixture into the molds. Pack it down firmly.

7. Let them dry for an hour and then tap the mold to release the bath bomb. Let the bombs sit out to dry for another hour before putting them away.

8. When you're ready to use one, all you have to do is throw it in the tub.

Bath Salts

These bath salts smell great and are guaranteed not to turn you into a zombie. While you can make these salts with just lavender oil, you're going to need a couple more types of essential oils for the best results. Adding the other two essential oils will make your bath absolutely divine.

<u>Ingredients</u>

½ cup Epsom salt

2 drops lavender essential oil

1 drop Roman chamomile essential oil (optional)

2 drops geranium essential oil (optional)

<u>Directions</u>

1. Stir the oil(s) into the ½ cup of Epsom salt.
2. Toss the salt into the tub while you're filling it up. By the time the tub is done filling, the salt and oil will have dissolved and the smell will be permeating the room.
3. Soak for 15 to 20 minutes, then get out of the tub and pat yourself dry.

Car Air Freshener

If you've ever bought one of those car air fresheners that are shaped like a pine tree, you've probably enjoyed the fresh pine scent for a few days to a week. One day you get to your car and find it's back to smelling like old shoes and that strawberry your son dropped behind the seat that you never found. If you're anything like I used to be, you spend a pretty penny keeping all of your vehicles smelling like a fresh forest . . . or a new car . . . or whatever fresh smell it is you prefer. With this tutorial, you won't have to buy an air freshener ever again. You can make your own rechargeable ones with this simple tutorial.

Ingredients

Sheet of wool felt.

Hole punch

Twine

10 to 20 drops of lavender oil

Directions

1. Cut the wool felt into whatever shape you like. If you prefer the pine trees, you can use that shape. If not, the world's the limit. I usually let my kids choose the shape the air freshener gets cut into. At least I used to. Until I hung an air freshener that I thought was a peach only to find out weeks later that my son had cut out a butt just to see if I'd hang it up. Now I'm the only one allowed to cut the felt.

2. Use the hole punch to punch a hole at the top.
3. Tie the string through the hole so it creates a loop you can use to hang the air freshener.
4. Add 10 to 20 drops of essential oil to the wool felt. The more drops you add, the stronger the scent will be. Don't underestimate how strong it will be in the confines of your car.
5. When the smell dissipates, recharge your air freshener by adding more essential oil to it.

NOTE: If you crave that pine fresh scent, you can buy pine essential oil. It smells great and is actually good for you, unlike those chemical fragrances the commercial air fresheners use.

Deodorant

If you're currently using store bought deodorant, I want you to take a close look at the ingredients listed on the label. There's some pretty bad stuff in there. Stuff you really shouldn't be applying to your body. With this recipe, you can make you own green deodorant at home that smells good and kills harmful bacterial on contact.

Ingredients

2 tablespoons cocoa butter

2 tablespoons coconut oil

1 tablespoon beeswax

3 tablespoons arrowroot powder

1 tablespoon baking soda

20 drops lavender essential oil

Directions

1. Add the cocoa butter, the coconut oil and the beeswax to a saucepan over low heat. Let them melt and stir them together.
2. Remove from heat and let cool for a few minutes until lukewarm.
3. Add the rest of the ingredients and stir them into the mixture.
4. Stir until mixture starts to thicken up.
5. Place into refrigerator until it gets hard.
6. Apply to armpits as needed.

Diffuser Recipes

So, you've bought a diffuser and some lavender essential oil. You've diffused lavender into every room in the house for months and it's starting to get a little boring. What can you do? Buy a few more oils and start making your own interesting blends for the diffuser. Here are a few to get you started.

Blend #1

2 drops cedar

4 drops lavender

3 drops spruce

Blend #2

6 drops lavender

2 drops rose

4 drops rosewood

1 drop ylang ylang

Blend #3

5 drops lavender

2 drops peppermint

3 drops Roman chamomile

Blend #4

4 drops lavender

3 drops rosemary

2 drops peppermint

Blend #5

4 drops bergamot

5 drops lavender

Blend #6

3 drops bergamot

4 drops lavender

3 drops spearmint

Blend #7

5 drops lavender

2 drops peppermint

2 drops tea tree oil

Blend #8

4 drops lavender

3 drops patchouli

Air Cleansing Blend

2 drops basil

2 drops Cedarwood

3 drops grapefruit

3 drops lavender

2 drops lemon

2 drops orange

Cold Buster Blend

5 drops eucalyptus

10 drops lavender

5 drops tea tree

Flu Buster Blend

2 drops cinnamon bark

3 drops eucalyptus

3 drops lavender

2 drops lemon

3 drops rosemary

Hangover Relief Blend

3 drops Juniper

5 drops lavender

3 drops rosemary

Headache Blend

3 drops lavender

3 drops lemon

2 drops grapefruit

2 drops peppermint

Insect Away Blend

4 drops citronella

3 drops eucalyptus

5 drops lavender

3 drops lemongrass

3 drop patchouli

Relaxation Blend

5 drops lavender

5 drops Roman chamomile

Romantic Blend

2 drops anise oil

1 drop black pepper

1 drop cinnamon

3 drops clary sage

3 drops lavender

3 drops rosewood

1 drop patchouli

Sleepy Time Blend

3 drops frankincense

5 drops lavender

2 drops Roman chamomile

2 drops German chamomile

Stress Relief Blend

5 drops lavender

5 drops lemongrass

3 drops ylang ylang

Hair Care Formula

Suffering from dry and damaged hair? Take care of it with this hair care oil blend. You're going to need basil essential oil to go along with your lavender oil for this recipe.

Ingredients

½ cup Jojoba oil

20 drops basil essential oil

20 drops lavender essential oil

Directions

1. Add ingredients to small bowl and mix until blended.
2. Add a small amount at a time to your hair and rub it into your hair and scalp.
3. Leave in for 15 to 20 minutes and wash out.

Homemade Lavender Scented Play Dough

Ever wanted to relive your childhood? Now you can with aromatherapy-grade play dough. Playing with dough will release the scent of lavender into the room and will help you relax. You can play with it with your kids before bedtime to help calm them down and get them ready for bed.

Ingredients

1 cup flour

1 cup warm water

½ cup salt

1 tablespoon canola oil

½ tablespoon cream of tartar sauce

3 drops of lavender essential oil

Food coloring (Kool-Aid packets will work in a pinch)

Directions

1. Add all of the ingredients except lavender oil and food coloring to a pot and stir them together over low heat.
2. Keep stirring until the dough starts to thicken.
3. Once dough starts to thicken and becomes hard to stir, turn off the heat.
4. Let cool until lukewarm and stir in essential oil and food coloring.

NOTE: You can separate out balls of dough and color them different colors, so you'll have a number of colors to choose from. You can also use different essential oils that have different qualities. Just make sure they aren't potential dermal irritants and make sure they're safe for kids if you plan on letting your kids play with them.

Face Mask

This face mask is designed to soothe the skin and help get rid of any inflammation. It works well for all skin types, but is tailor-made for those with redness due to rosacea. It requires the purchase of two additional essential oils. Rose and chamomile. Rose oil can be a bit on the expensive side, but a little oil goes a long way. All you need is a few drops for this recipe.

Ingredients

¼ cup plain unsweetened yogurt

1 ½ tablespoons honey

5 drops lavender essential oil

2 drops Roman chamomile essential oil

2 drops rose essential oil

Directions

1. Add all ingredients to a small bowl and stir together until blended.
2. Wash your face and spread the blend over your face, avoiding the eyes.
3. Let sit for 20 minutes and wash off with lukewarm water.

Lip Balm

I've been making my own lip balm for a couple years now and it's so much better than the stuff you get from the store. It's inexpensive to make and feels so much better on your lips. Best of all, it's easy to make and almost impossible to get wrong.

Ingredients

¼ cup beeswax, grated

¼ cup coconut oil

¼ cup Jojoba oil

2 teaspoons vitamin E oil

20 drops lavender essential oil

Directions

1. Add the beeswax, coconut oil and Jojoba oil to a saucepan and melt over low heat, stirring frequently.
2. Add the vitamin E oil and stir it in.
3. Remove from heat and let cool until lukewarm. Stir in the lavender essential oil.
4. Pour into containers and let sit in the open until the lip balm solidifies.

Massage Oil

Adding lavender oil to a massage oil blend gives you the benefit of the massage, plus the therapeutic qualities of the lavender oil. It's a win-win situation. This combination is sure to help you relax.

Ingredients

1 cup avocado oil

1 tablespoon Shea butter

1 cup sunflower oil

25 drops lavender essential oil

Directions

1. Add all ingredients except for the lavender oil to a saucepan on low heat. Warm it up and stir it together.
2. Remove the saucepan from the heat and let the mixture cool for a couple minutes until lukewarm.
3. Stir the lavender oil into the mix.

Moisturizing Coconut Lavender Skin Cream

This recipe is ideal for those who have dry, cracked skin. The coconut oil moisturizes your skin, while the lavender oil promotes healing and knocks down any inflammation you may have. Did I mention it smells great? Package this in a nice container and it makes for a great gift.

Ingredients

3 cups coconut oil

30 drops lavender essential oil

Natural purple coloring (optional)

Directions

4. Place the solid coconut oil into a mixing bowl. If your coconut oil is in liquid form, cool it down a bit and it should solidify.
5. Use a mixer set on high to whip the coconut oil until light and fluffy.
6. Add the lavender essential oil and blend it in.
7. Store the skin cream in an airtight container in a cool, dark place until you're ready to use it.

Soothing Spray

This soothing spray has been a life-saver. It's helped me calm down and relax when I'm feeling particularly stressed out. I'm almost embarrassed to admit I've used it on my kids from time-to-time when they're especially rambunctious. It calms them down enough for me to get them under control. To use this spray, all you have to do is put the recipe below in a spray bottle and spray three to four sprays of fine mist into the air. Instant relaxation.

Ingredients

½ cup water

15 drops lavender essential oil

15 drops rosemary essential oil

Directions

1. Add oils and water to a spray bottle.
2. Shake it up.
3. Spray 3 to 4 sprays of fine mist into the air.

Waterless Hand Cleanser

Looking for an all-natural alternative to the chemical-filled soaps you've been buying in the store? This hand cleanser gets your hands clean and makes them smell great in the process. The base recipe uses just lavender and tea tree essential oil. If you're feeling adventurous, try adding other essential oils to the mix to create interesting and complex fragrances.

Ingredients

½ cup aloe Vera gel

20 drops lavender essential oil

5 drops tea tree essential oil (optional)

Directions

8. Stir the oils into the aloe Vera gel until incorporated.
9. Add the mixture to a squirt bottle and dispense on your hands when you want to clean them.
10. Rub your hands together until the mixture soaks in.

Did You Enjoy This Book?

I hope you enjoyed reading about lavender essential oil and its many uses as much as I enjoyed writing about it. Thanks for purchasing (or downloading) this book. If you're interested in expanding your knowledge of essential oils, you can check out my comprehensive book of essential oils and their many uses and applications. Here's a link you can use to buy it from Amazon.com:

http://www.amazon.com/Aromatherapy-Essential-Oils-Handbook-ebook/dp/B00BECCJXY/

If you have any questions or comments, feel free to drop me a line at the following e-mail address:

mike_rashelle@yahoo.com